ST BARTHOLOMEW'S HOSPITAL
IN PEACE AND WAR

ST BARTHOLOMEW'S HOSPITAL IN PEACE AND WAR

THE REDE LECTURE
1915

by

NORMAN MOORE, M.D.

Fellow of the Royal College of Physicians
Honorary Fellow of St Catharine's College
Consulting Physician to St Bartholomew's Hospital

Cambridge :
at the University Press
1915

CAMBRIDGE
UNIVERSITY PRESS

32 Avenue of the Americas, New York NY 10013-2473, USA

Cambridge University Press is part of the University of Cambridge.

It furthers the University's mission by disseminating knowledge in the pursuit of
education, learning and research at the highest international levels of excellence.

www.cambridge.org
Information on this title: www.cambridge.org/9781107418868

First published 1915
First paperback edition 2014

A catalogue record for this publication is available from the British Library

ISBN 978-1-107-41886-8 Paperback

ST BARTHOLOMEW'S HOSPITAL
IN PEACE AND WAR

MORE than forty years ago, after kneeling
at the feet of a venerable man who occupied
the seat in which you, Mr Vice-Chancellor, are
now enthroned and receiving from him my first
degree, I left the precincts of the University
and at once began the study of medicine in
the hospital of St Bartholomew in London,
with which I have ever since been connected,
and for which as long as I live I shall retain a
veneration scarcely less than that which every
son of this University has for Alma Mater
Cantabrigia.

My work caused me to live for twenty-one
years in the hospital within the jurisdiction of
the Lord Mayor and Aldermen and to traverse
every part of the City of London. I became

ST BARTHOLOMEW'S HOSPITAL

familiar with the outline of St Paul's against the sky illuminated by sunrise and often felt the morning breeze which plays across its west front as if in perpetual memory of Richard of Beaumes[1] who made an open space before the cathedral by purchasing and pulling down the houses which in his time stood close to it. I saw the streets crowded all day long with moving men and vehicles for the most part started on their way by the commerce of England,

> By which remotest regions are allied:
> Which makes one city of the universe,
> Where some may gain and all may be supplied.

By day too many men are going to and fro for any study except that of the actual moment or for any meditation except perhaps some passing thoughts on the Mare Liberum of Grotius as the true explanation of the

[1] William of Malmesbury.

scene or the Vision of Mirzah as the natural moralization upon it. I came also to know well the charm of the almost deserted streets in moonlight. In that time of stillness their vistas, their directions, their names and the titles of their buildings seem to set forth the history of past centuries. Now and then great bursts of flame with the crackling of combustion would alarm the night, and on a sudden the sky was filled with floating fragments of red-hot gold lace or a stream of blazing oil flowed into the river. The violence of the scene brought up at once the memory of the time when the whole city was destroyed by fire:

> Now down the narrow streets it swiftly came,
> And widely opening did on both sides prey:
> This benefit we sadly owe the flame,
> If only ruin must enlarge our way.

I had seen the bones of men who died of the plague of 1348–1357, exposed to view in the pits where they had been buried in land purchased from St Bartholomew's, and once walking along the line of streets which traverses the city from west to east, close to the site of the house of Sir Richard Blackmore, physician and epic writer, I heard from a man who had just visited a case the news of the appearance of plague after an interval of more than two hundred years.

The city was a scene of the utmost activity of peace. Martial display seemed no part of what it had to show. At that time the vessels of war which now sail round St Paul's were unknown. The loud whirr of the aeroplane was never heard. No foe had tried to traverse the sky and to find out

> His uncouth way, or spread his airy flight,
> Upborne with indefatigable wings
> Over the vast abrupt, ere he arrive
> The happy isle.

When any regiment appeared, except one

raised in the city, it halted to unfix bayonets at the boundary of the liberties, but this was a rare occurrence, and the only soldiers often seen were a detachment of foot guards who marched every evening to the Bank of England and quickly entering a narrow door guarded many millions of treasure during the night. Yet the city was once surrounded by a wall which has been worn away by the advance of commerce and not by the assaults of war, and the course of which may still be followed. One bastion and a few fragments are still standing, and such names as London Wall and Old Bailey guide the eye to its alignment, while the names of its seven gates, Newgate, Ludgate, Aldersgate, Cripplegate, Moorgate, Aldgate, Bishopsgate, remain to testify to the ancient completeness of the enclosure. The ditch outside the wall is filled up and buried so deep that except in the name of one street it scarcely comes before the population of to-day, but once when some long-suppressed springs were allowed to burst forth in the course of building operations I saw the waters extended from the wall to nearly the ancient breadth of the ditch near Newgate.

The appearance of the greatest person of the present in the city, the Lord Mayor, soon became familiar to me. I saw him driving about in his gilt coach with mace and sword protruding from the windows, and on the day of his installation proceeding round the ward of which he was alderman or on some other day waiting at the edge of the liberties of the city where by Temple Bar he dismounted and humbly surrendered to his sovereign the sword of state, thus showing whence his authority was derived. In time it became my duty to call on this potentate and upon

each of the aldermen and certain of the
members of the council and thus I respectfully
viewed the corporation. Ancient as the office
of the Mayor was, it was yet by seventy years
of less antiquity than the hospital into which
I entered when I came from Cambridge by a
path which had certainly been trodden by
men who remembered St Anselm as Archbishop of Canterbury.

The citizen of the remote past held in
greatest honour within the city I learned to
be Thomas Beket, Archbishop of Canterbury,
since his figure was for more than four
centuries to be seen upon the common seal
appended to deeds. In the oldest impressions
he is represented in his pontifical vestments
seated upon a throne in the arch of heaven,
giving his benediction to the city beneath
while a group of laymen kneel on his left and
of clerks on his right. On the later seal he is

seated beside St Paul each under an ornate canopy. That London had given birth to him was counted one of its greatest glories. When he was slain in his cathedral the hospital had been in existence for forty-six years and the year of his canonization was the fiftieth of its growth. A copy of a brief in which he mentions St Bartholomew's Hospital is preserved in its cartulary. He confirms in their privileges "that place in Smithfield in which the church of the canons is built and the hospital house of that church" exactly as they were granted by King Henry I. King Henry in his charter, of which more than one ancient copy exists, granted, with certain reservations, complete freedom to the Prior and canons of the church and to the poor of the hospital of the church and confirmed the grant in a further charter in 1133.

The hospital occupies the whole of one side of Smithfield, an open space mentioned in the life of St Thomas of Canterbury and in the book of William, son of Stephen his secretary, and very often in English history since. How the hospital came to be there is related in the manuscript called "Liber fundacionis," which belonged to the Priory of St Bartholomew, and later stood in the ninth place on the second shelf under the bust of Vespasian in Sir Robert Cotton's library. It is a copy made in the reign of Richard II of a book composed in the time of Henry II. The pilgrimage to Rome of Rahere, the founder, his visit to St Paul's outside the walls of Rome, his fever, his vision, his vow to found a hospital outside the wall of London, his further vow to found a priory of Augustinian canons and his success in the fulfilment of both vows with the aid of Henry I and of

Richard of Beaumes, Bishop of London, are well known from this book.

The pathway through the Smithfield gate by which I entered the hospital for the first time in 1869 was the entrance in the time of Rahere, who died on September 20, 1145. Within the gate on the site of the present church of St Bartholomew the Less, stood a chapel dedicated with the hospital to the Exaltation of the Holy Cross. It is curious how difficult is the imposition of a name. The history of Rahere's vision and vow to St Bartholomew was so well known that in spite of formal dedication to the Exaltation of the Holy Cross, the hospital was always called St Bartholomew's during the Middle Ages.

"Be it known to you all," says Andrew Buckerell when starting on a pilgrimage in the last quarter of the twelfth century, "that for the love of God and for the welfare of the souls of Stephen my father and Sabella my mother, and of my own soul and that of Ydonea my wife, and those of our children and of all our friends, that I have granted and given in the days of my prosperity and before starting on my pilgrimage six shillings of rent to the hospital of St Bartholomew and to the brethren of the same."

A hundred years later, between 1281 and 1285, Geoffrey Gykel granted to the Master, brethren and sisters of St Bartholomew of Smethefend, a form which occasionally occurs for Smithfield, "a croft in the parish of Donton which stretches in length from the land of the monks of Bec to the royal way which goes from London towards Reile." A bull of Pope Alexander III (1159–1181) is addressed "dilectis filiis preceptori et fratribus hospitalis domus sancti Bartholomei de Smedhefeld," and one of Pope Lucius III in 1183 "dilectis filiis Alano presbytero procuratori hospitalis domus de Smethfulde eiusque fratribus tam presentibus quam futuris canonice instituendis in perpetuum." Pope Clement V in February, 1306, directs the abbot of Holy Cross at Waltham in the diocese of London to investigate a question about the property of the master and brethren of the hospital of St Bartholomew.

On January 14, 1391, as is recorded in an original indenture, John Harmesthorp, master of the hospital of St Katharine by the Tower of London and the brethren and sisters thereof, received from William Wakeryng, master of the hospital of St Bartholomew next Smithfield of the same city, and its brethren and sisters, twenty shillings sterling in acquittance of all arrears of a quit rent of three shillings.

The list of Masters of the hospital written

in the reign of Henry VI is headed "Nomina Magistrorum Hospitalis Sancti Bartholomei nuncupati et in honore Exaltacionis Sancte Crucis fundati." There is, however, no need to quote other examples since its own seals and all charters call the hospital St Bartholomew's throughout the Middle Ages.

King Henry VIII at first proposed that it should be called "The Hospital of St Bartholomew in West Smithfeilde by the foundation of our Lord King Henry the 8th In the Honour of the holye and undivide Trinity," but afterwards ordered that it should be called "The house of the Poor in West Smithfield in the Suburbs of the City of London of King Henry VIII's foundation." This is the form used in Acts of Parliament and in leases sealed at the Guildhall, but in daily life the hospital has been St Bartholomew's ever since Henry VIII as it was before his alterations.

The present stately quadrangle of the hospital was built by James Gibbs, the architect of the churches of St Martin's in the Fields and St Mary le Strand in London, of the Radcliffe library at Oxford and of the fellows' buildings of King's College. One of its staircases was decorated by Hogarth, in memory of his birth in the neighbourhood, with great canvases depicting the Pool of Bethesda and the parable of the Good Samaritan, while in the same pile of buildings there hangs in an office a gilded oak chandelier carved by John Freke, surgeon to the hospital, one of the first English writers on electricity, a friend of Fielding and twice mentioned in *Tom Jones*. Thus the eighteenth century in which the mediaeval hospital was replaced by a modern building was every day plain to be seen by a student working within it.

The frequent mention of Harvey by phy-

sicians and surgeons and lecturers of the staff,
the indication of the residence of Sir Thomas
Bodley within the hospital by his wife's tomb
in the church, a portrait of Sir Nicholas
Rainton, President of the Hospital, who was
sent to the Tower in May, 1640, for resisting
an unlawful attempt at taxation by refusing
to make lists of inhabitants of wards able to
contribute £50 or more to a loan for the
service of the Crown; the portrait of Martin
Bond, a treasurer, whose building of Aldgate
was watched by Ben Jonson, and Bond's
inkstand every day upon the office table, all
these brought back the seventeenth century.
The charter under which the hospital is
governed and by which it is connected with
the City of London, the words of the charges
delivered to the several officers on their
appointment were perpetual reminders of the
sixteenth century, of King Henry VIII and

King Edward VI, and of the many years during which Dr Caius lived in St Bartholomew's and had his treatise on the Sweating Sickness printed in the neighbouring cloister of the Franciscans by Richard Grafton, the author of the chronicle, and acting treasurer of St Bartholomew's, who narrowly escaped an untimely fate since he printed the proclamation of Queen Jane at the beginning of her nine days' reign.

The fifteenth century and all the other centuries up to the time of our founder Rahere were brought to mind by the ancient cartulary of the hospital written in the reign of Henry VI and containing a copy of every royal or private charter and of every papal bull belonging at that time to St Bartholomew's.

Books of this kind received names from the imagination they aroused, from their contents or from their external features.

The terms Domesday, Redituarium, Boss book, were equally applied to them in the Middle Ages, and at the present day they are most often called Cartularies. The first term owed its origin, like the Conqueror's record of England, to the great book of the Last Judgment:

> Liber scriptus proferetur
> In quo totum continetur
> Unde mundus judicetur.

The last term was derived from the metal bosses projecting from and fastening the leather which covered its oak boards. All three names are applied on different occasions to the St Bartholomew's book. It was written by John Cok, one of the eight brethren of the hospital in the reign of King Henry VI, and has remained there ever since.

The mediaeval writer when he was both an author and a scribe generally left traces of his individuality in his manuscripts: how each was begun, how ended, why undertaken, when he was fatigued, when depressed, when joyful. Cok followed this custom, and from passages in the cartulary of St Bartholomew's something may be learned of its writer. He was born in 1392. A house in Wood street yielded a quit rent to the hospital, and when Cok mentions this in the list of rents he says: "and in which tenement and in which time I John Cok who compiled this rental and wrote it out was then and there apprenticed in the first year of King Henry V." On the last leaf, in a summary of the reigns of the kings of England, he records another event of his youth: "In the year 1413 on the ninth day of the month of April, which day was Passion Sunday, and a very rainy day, the coronation of Henry V took place at Westminster, which coronation I brother John Cok beheld and have recorded for the refreshing of memory."

Thus did Cok see under the vault of Westminster Abbey

> Harry the king, Bedford and Exeter,
> Warwick and Talbot, Salisbury and Gloucester,

those great warriors of five hundred years ago whose fellow-countrymen, and among them so many members of this University, are at this day engaging with equal courage, and for a better reason, a fiercer and more numerous foe on the same field of war, and will at last attain a still greater victory. Talbot was a tenant of St Bartholomew's and his town house was in Smithfield. It was called Tiptoft's hospice after the Speaker of the House of Commons of 1406, who occupied it before Talbot.

Cok learned artistic writing and drawing during his apprenticeship. He seems to have retained a pleasant memory of his goldsmith days, for in an illuminated initial he is represented in a goldsmith's habit, a red gown and black cap. I wish that in the many ornate initials which are clearly from his hand he had left a sketch of Wood street as he knew it or of some parts of its long narrow course. A few features of his time are discoverable at this day. Near Cheapside, on the west side of Wood street, the unused cemetery of the church of St Peter in Chepe is one such. Further north, on the east side of the street, the church of St Alban, built by Wren, is the successor of one which was standing there in the reign of Henry II and marked the connection between Wood street and the great abbey of St Alban's. Stow was wrong when he attributed the name of the street to the family of a sheriff of 1491, Thomas Wood. An agreement between Symon, abbot of St Alban's, and St Bartholomew's Hospital, of which I have seen the original, was written in the mastership of Adam le Mercer, which ended in 1167, the year in which Symon was chosen abbot on May 30, so that the document belongs to one of the later months of that year. Its subject is a tenement in this Wood street. "This is an agreement between abbot Symon and the church of St Albans and the Hospital of St Bartholomew in Smithfield of London. Namely that the brethren of that hospital shall hold by perpetual right of the church of St Alban the whole tenement which Gervase the clerk has held of the church of St Alban in Wode street of London returning thence every year by the hand of him who should be warden and procurator of the hospital to the church of St Alban four shillings at two terms. Namely two at Easter and two at Michaelmas. The brethren of the aforesaid hospital shall besides hold the tenement which Henry le

Estreis held in Wode street of the church of St Alban: paying yearly thence to the said church three shillings at the above mentioned terms. Namely at each eighteenpence. These being witnesses Adam le mercer: Martin: Hugh of Clovilla: Terric bette: Michael of Valenciennes: Martin the Lorrainer: Race of Merideizre: William the esquire: Alan of Chauz: William the chaplain: Alan the clerk: Symon son of Gaufrid: Albert the lorimer." The word chirographum at one side is cut in two. The abbey of St Alban's had one half, St Bartholomew's the other. The seal "Sigillum Sancti Albani Anglorum Protomartiris" is curiously attached at the side. The first witness, Adam le mercer, was master of the hospital. Michael of Valenciennes was for several years alderman of the ward of Aldersgate.

Cok copied this charter. So it is easy to

see that in 1413 he knew Wood street, Cheapside, as well as we do. A man of to-day who
walks down it, unconcerned with the rushing
crowd of commerce, perhaps thinks of Words-
worth, who had visited it twice, and who,
though he retained a confused recollection of
its geographical position, has touched the
street with the wand of poetry:

At the corner of Wood street when daylight appears
There's a thrush that sings loud—it has sung for three years;
Poor Susan has passed by the spot and has heard
In the silence of morning the song of the bird.

'Tis a note of enchantment: what ails her? she sees
A mountain ascending, a vision of trees,
Bright volumes of vapour through Lothbury glide,
And a river flows on through the vale of Cheapside.

A tree at the end of the street marks the site
of the church of St Peter in Chepe.

Cok, it is easy to imagine, repeated to
himself as he walked there the line of Colum-
banus:

Aurum flamma probat: homines tentatio justos

or some verses reciting the skill and virtues of St Dunstan, the patron of his craft.

When he became deep in the business affairs of St Bartholomew's, Wood street had another association for Cok. Out of it a narrow lane, now called Fell street, leads into Mugwell (now Monkswell) street, and the south side of that lane, then part of Cripple-gate street, of which only one side had been built, had been the land of Thomas Fitz Thomas, the mayor, and his adherents, Richard Trissell and William Ardern, who had sided with Simon de Montfort and lost all at Evesham. The land was granted to John de Muscegros in the forty-ninth year of Henry III under his great seal. The witnesses, many of them, were on the royal side at Lewes or at Evesham. Hugh le bigot escaped capture at the end of the defeat of Lewes and fought at Evesham. Philip Basset, Roger of Clifford and Roger of

Leyburn fought at Lewes. Robert Walerand
fought at Evesham. John de Muscegros in
1274 made over the land to Sir Bartholomew
de Bryan, sometime constable of the Tower
of London. Bryan bequeathed it to William
of Gravele, who sold it in 1286 to William de
Marisco, who sold it in 1298 to Theobald of
Merk, who in 1315 sold it to his son William
of Herle, and he in 1322 to William of Perten-
hale, citizen and corn merchant. This citizen,
by a will proved February 21, 1348, bequeathed the land to his wife and two children
and after them to St Bartholomew's Hospital.
His daughter Joan was the survivor, and she
was admitted a sister of St Bartholomew's.
She was still living in 1386, and at her death
the hospital became possessed of the estate,
which was regranted to it by King Henry VIII.
Till a few years ago an old warehouse with a
doorway made of the jaws of a Greenland

whale gave it a picturesque aspect, though there were no architectural features to carry the mind back to the series of ancient owners, or to the Barons' war, the battle of Evesham, or the ruin of Thomas, son of Thomas, son of Richard, Mayor of London.

To return to Cok's life as it may be extracted from the cartulary. In 1418 he came into the employment of Robert Newton, who lived near the chapel of St Andrew in the hospital and was a member of the foundation and probably the redituarius or rentar. Newton had been appointed Master by Richard Clifford, Bishop of London, on June 13, 1413, and resigned on May 31, 1415. He was succeeded on July 3, 1415, by John Bury, who died September 28, 1417. John White, who had been rector of the church of St Michael Paternoster for eleven years, was then, after profession as a brother of the hospital on December 23, 1417, appointed Master in January, 1418, and held office till February 13, 1423. It was in 1420, during White's mastership, that Cok became a brother. He took part in the next election of a master. The chapter of the hospital met on March 2, 1423, and 'per viam Spiritus Sancti' acclaimed as master, John Wakering alias Blackberd, one of the brethren. Wakering held office for forty years. How Cok admired him is shown by a note written in the cartulary after the account of the election : "and I brother John Cok lived throughout his mastership, who put down in writing all his famous works. For the wondrous acuteness of his extraordinary discretion ought to be recorded."

Cok succeeded to the office of rentar, which Newton had held when Cok was first employed by him. Cok's excellence in the art of writing, his accuracy and his love of St Bartholomew's Hospital fitted him in every way for this post. The writing of the cartulary became the chief work of his life. He calls the book a Rental: Redituarium. It is made up of 636 leaves of vellum and contains copies of 1433 charters, as well as a record of all rents due to the hospital and other information such as a list of masters and a glossary of terms. Wakeryng vacated the mastership on November 16, 1466, but Cok worked on under the new master, John Needham, who was elected on December 3, 1466. The last words written by John Cok are at the end of a beautiful transcript of a bull of Pope Nicholas V:

"Written by brother John Cok in the evening of his life Anno Domini 1468 on whose soul may God have mercy."

The end of his life thus coincided with the

beginning of that of Sir Robert Rede, chief
justice of the Common Pleas, the munificent
founder of the present lecture and of other
endowments in this University and in particular colleges here.

Cok's cartulary, with some aid from other
manuscripts, such as the cartulary of the
Benedictine nuns of Clerkenwell, the cartulary
of the lepers of St Giles, and the hairy book
of St Paul's, explains the parts of the city
lying near St Bartholomew's or connected
with it.

At the present day the side of Smithfield
opposite to the hospital is occupied by
modern warehouses and other places of business, but the opening of Hosier lane was there
in the time of Cok as it is to-day and the
tower of St Sepulchre's Church was then, as
now, to be seen to the south-west of Smithfield. To the north an Early English door

is all that is left of the west front of the
church of St Bartholomew's priory as it was
known to Cok. St Sepulchre's is named in
the earliest existing original charter in which
the hospital is mentioned. In this document
Rahere grants to Hagno the clerk, an Augustinian canon, the church of St Sepulchre.
Hagno is to pay fifty shillings every year for
the use of the canons and of the poor in the
hospital. The charter is dated in the year
1137, the second of the rule of King Stephen
in England, and is witnessed by Haco the
dean and sixteen other witnesses.

St Sepulchre's Church is at the top of a
slope which declines from Newgate to the
Fleet river, which at the present day flows
underground into the Thames at Blackfriars.
From the church looking east you can see the
straight line of fortification, the Old Bailey,
and over the ancient site of the New Gate

into the intramural part of the ward of Faringdon and as far as the church of St Mary le Bow, Sancta Maria de Arcubus, in the ward of Chepe. Looking west, the Holborn Viaduct now conceals the valley of the Fleet, beyond which on the southern side of the way stands the church of St Andrew. From this church Holborn slopes uphill to the granite pillars which mark the position of the Bars which were the boundaries of the Liberties of the City and which in the reign of John showed the western limit of the great ward of Joce son of Peter. In a charter witnessed by Henry Fitz Eilwin, the first Mayor of London, and ten other witnesses, Joce son of Peter granted three shillings of quit rent from some land in the parish of St Martin Ludgate to St Bartholomew's Hospital, "and it is to be known," he says in the charter, "that the aforesaid brethren of the hospital of

St Bartholomew have granted to me that annually on the morrow of the feast of All Saints, namely on the day of the commemoration of all the faithful departed, they shall spend and give away the aforesaid three shillings in the sustenance of the poor."

Holborn is a very ancient name. A street with a name which also goes back into the beginnings of the history of the city leads south from the church of St Andrew in Holborn to the parish of St Bride where it opens into Fleet street. This is Shoe lane, a street so old that the origin of its name has been entirely forgotten. It has nothing to do with the material of the cordwainer or the work of the tacunarius. The original form of its name occurs in several ancient charters: as in that of Walter the chaplain, procurator of the sick of the hospital of St Giles to Maurice the parmentar. It probably belongs to the first years of the thirteenth century, and begins: "Know all present and to come that I Walter the chaplain, procurator of the sick, of the hospital of St Giles outside London and the brethren and sisters of the same place by the advice and consent of Andrew Bukerel and William Hardel then guardians of that hospital," grant to Maurice the maker of fur robes part of our land in the parish of St Brigid the virgin "in vico que vocatur Solande." The hospital was one of lepers, so that it needed guardians to act for it in the outer world. The seventh of eight witnesses of another original charter of an early year of King John gives the original name without the addition of 'street.' The grantor is Robert de Lalieflonde, warden of the gaol of Flete:

"Know men present and to come that I Robert de Lalieflonde, warden of the gaol of

Flete, for the welfare of my soul and that of my wife and those of my children and of my father and my mother and my ancestors have given and granted and by this my charter confirmed to God and to the brethren of the Hospital of St Bartholomew's of London, the passage over Fleet water for all ships which carry the goods of the aforesaid Hospital, both going in and coming out, without either custom or exaction, in free, pure and perpetual alms for ever. So that neither I Robert de Lalieflonde, nor my heirs nor any through us shall set up any claim on these aforesaid ships. And because I wish that the gift and concession and confirmation of the present charter shall be settled and unbroken I confirm it by the apposition of this my seal.

"These being witnesses: Robert of Wincestre: Henry of St Albans: Richard of Wincestre: Reginald le Bucher: Simon of the bridge of Fleet: Robert reidevele: Alexander of Solanda: Warin the parchiminer: and many others."

The same Robert in another original charter granted to St Bartholomew's certain land between the land of the abbot of Cirencester and the Fleet river and on the other part between the land of William of Tonbridge and the lane leading from the Fleet river to the street of Solanda at an annual rent of two shillings sterling.

In 1283 land in the street is mentioned as "in vico de Solande." Cok, in the reign of Henry VI, writes the word "Sholane." The word *solanda* does not occur in Du Cange, but appears, according to the learned editor of the Domesday of St Paul's, to mean a prebendal farm. These charters show that Shoe lane is merely a mistaken etymology of solanda. The prebendal lands on this side of the cathedral began with Holborn and went on to Portpoole and Kentish Town. It was perhaps to the prebend of Holborn that this particular solanda belonged.

The grant of Robert de Lalieflonde was a valuable benefaction to the hospital, for by the Fleet river the brethren could bring up their rents paid in kind in Essex, by water to the landing place of the knights hospitallers somewhere near the present station of the Metropolitan Railway in Faringdon street. Lalieflonde's device was a boar's head with large tusks, a not inappropriate representation of the ferocity of prison life in his time. The Fleet river became a mere sewer:

> The king of dykes than whom no sluice of mud
> With deeper sable blots the silver flood.

Since Pope's time it has been shut up in a tubular dungeon which conducts it under the pavement of Faringdon street and Bridge street to its old opening into the Thames, as if to remind it of all the unhappiness it had passed by in the Gaol of Flete from the time when Robert de Lalieflonde watched the ships passing up it with corn for St Bartholomew's Hospital brought from Little Wakering creek to the days when the oppressions wrought upon those imprisoned for debt in the prison excited the indignation of Charles Dickens and stirred him to use his wonderful pen for its destruction.

It is possible that some old man who remembered the death of Harold and the foundation of Battle Abbey on the field where England was lost and won may have ended his days in St Bartholomew's, but the first recorded warriors known to the hospital were the witnesses of King Henry I's charter, men who soon after took part in the wars of Stephen: Roger the burly bishop of Sarum, who stood siege in Devizes castle; Stephen, himself at the time of the charter earl of Mortaign; Alberic de Vere, Milo of Gloucester, Pagan FitzJohn, Robert de Curci, who were all present in 1133 when the king's seal was affixed. The next soldiers who knew of the hospital and its patients had taken part in a more memorable contest: that which ended in the grant of Magna Carta.

Lord Chatham was speaking as a student of human nature, and not of the details of thirteenth century history, when he compared the iron barons of the Great Charter, as he called them, to the silken barons of later times. "Their virtues," he said, "were rude and uncultivated but they were great and sincere. Their understandings were as little polished as their manners, but they had hearts to distinguish right from wrong, they had heads to distinguish truth from falsehood, they understood the rights of humanity and they had the spirit to maintain them."

Such was the traditional basis of our statute book, and among the great men whose influence or whose swords led to its grant several were acquainted with the hospital of St Bartholomew. Among the venerable fathers and noble men named in the preamble of the charter as those by whose advice it was granted, Joscelin Bishop of Bath and Glastonbury, William Earl of Salisbury, and Robert son of Walter were benefactors of St Bartholomew's Hospital. Bishop Joscelin granted to the Master and brethren on August 1, 1220, a tithe of the sheaves of the church land of the parish of Hinton St George and half of the tithes of all other sheaves belonging to the church and the whole tithe of hay from the domain of Robert of Barneville and two acres of land in that vill.

William Longespée, Earl of Salisbury, who was present when the foundation stone of Salisbury Cathedral was laid and who died on March 7, 1226, gave to the hospital by his will eight oxen; Robert son of Walter, son of Robert, who led the barons into London on May 17, 1215, gave to the brethren of the hospital a way in and out of his marsh of Burnham from their marsh called le Suthwale, and gave them leave to ride or drive or lead flocks by these ways.

Richard of Muntfichet, the last but one of the twenty-five barons, was commanded by Henry III in 1229 to deliver to the Master of St Bartholomew's Hospital or to someone nominated by him six leafless oaks for the hospital fire.

Serlo the mercer, another of the barons, was Mayor of London in 1214–1215. The first mayor emerges from the obscurity of the

past on a subscription list, that for collecting
King Richard Coeur de Lion's ransom in
April 1193, and Serlo, the third mayor, appears
as one of the maintainers of English liberty
in Magna Carta—two functions happily main-
tained throughout English history by their
successors. Serlo had two periods of office
as mayor: 1214–1215 and 1217–1222. In
his time important charters in the City of
London which did not concern the church
were usually witnessed, in order, by the
mayor, the sheriffs, the alderman in whose
ward the land concerned lay, then by several
citizens of position more or less in the order
of their seniority in the city and often finally
by the scribe who wrote the charter and the
bedell of the ward. Serlo several times
appears as a first witness in documents
relating to St Bartholomew's, as in a charter
of John son of Galfrid Bocointe, who granted

five shillings of quit rent, from his capital messuage in the parish of St Andrew at Holborn, towards the lamp of the hospital. The Bocointes were a great family in London during the latter half of the twelfth century and the first two-thirds of the thirteenth. Three of them in the reign of Henry II, namely, John, William son of Sabelina, and Hersent wife of Gaufrid of St Loy, granted to Adam, the master, and the brethren of the hospital certain land on the side of Smithfield to right and left of the chapel of the hospital, now the church of St Bartholomew the Less. The brethren gave three talents of gold— these were the large gold coins of the Emperor of the East—in gersumam, that is, on con- clusion of the bargain, one to each of the three Bocointes. As Adam ceased to be master in 1168, the grant is earlier than that year. Henry FitzAilwin, afterwards mayor,

is one of the witnesses, and is followed by
Alulf, son of Fromund. This Alulf had three
descendants whose names are to be found
together in very many charters of the first
twenty-two years of the thirteenth century
in London: Constantine son of Alulf, Ernulf
Constantine's brother, and young Constantine.
The last was son of Alicia, daughter of Alulf
and wife of Richard of Heregird. These
three names always occur in the same order,
and after August, 1222, they never appear
again, for at that time the two Constantines
were, without trial, hanged. This grave in-
justice and inexcusable breach of Magna
Carta enables us to determine the approximate
date of the very many charters which the sons
of Alulf and their nephew witnessed. Their
ancestor was Fromund, an alderman of the
reign of Henry II, who had two sons, Alulf
and Pentecost. The latter lived in the parish

of St Nicholas ad macellas, near St Bartholomew's, where Pentecost lane long preserved
his name. Alulf, as a charter in the cartulary
of the nuns of Clerkenwell shows, had a stone
house and land in the parish of All Hallows,
Bread street. Four of his sons are mentioned
in this charter: Constantine, Fromund, Adam
and Arnulf, and one daughter, Alicia, married
to Richard Herierd, justiciar of the King.
Her son is always called young Constantine.
Constantine, son of Alulf, was at one time an
alderman, as is shown in another charter of
St Mary of Clerkenwell, and was sheriff in
1197. Louis of France, afterwards Louis VIII,
entered London on June 2, 1216, and was
received as a friend by many of the inhabitants, ecclesiastics as well as laymen. He
afterwards took the Tower of London and
many other castles and stayed for more than
a year. When he left in the autumn of 1217

a party in his favour still remained in the city. During his stay, Juliana, relict of Alan Balun, granted four shillings of quit rent to St Bartholomew's from a shop opposite the church of St Michael, Queenhithe. She declares that she has affixed her seal on the Nativity of St John the Baptist next after the first coming of Lord Louis, eldest son of the King of France, into England. Her grant is witnessed by three chaplains of the hospital, Bartholomew, Thomas and William, then by the family group, Constantine son of Alulf, Ernald Rufus and young Constantine. Michael of St Helena, John Herlicun, John Viel and John of Valencins are the other witnesses. John Herlicun, like the sons and grandson of Alulf, certainly belonged to the French party.

An agreement between Hugh, master of St Bartholomew's, and Reginald, the chaplain, son of Henry le Perer, about a house in the parish of St Martin, Ludgate, is dated at the end of this period of French invasion. The house was to be held for the eight years after the feast of St Michael next following the death of the Count de la Perche at Lincoln. The count's death had recently occurred.

Nichola of Camville was holding the castle of Lincoln for King Henry III, and William le Marechal came to its relief. The army of the king had broken down the gates and was fighting in the streets of the city. "They rushed in close ranks upon the Count of Perche," says Matthew Paris, "surrounding him on all sides and the weight of fighting was turned against him." The narrative of the count's death in *L'Histoire de Guillaume le Maréchal* which M. Paul Meyer discovered and edited, is probably the account given by the marshal himself to his household and friends: the marshal seized the reins of the

count's horse; but at this time he had
already received his mortal wound by a sword
thrust through his vizor by Sire Reinal Croc,
yet had strength to raise his sword with both
hands and to strike three blows which dented
the marshal's helmet. The count fell off his
horse. His helmet was loosened and it was
seen that he was dead. Louis had gone in
the early autumn of 1217. It had been agreed
that those in the city who had supported him,
except some ecclesiastics, should be un-
molested. The final destruction of the French
party took place in 1222 and followed a
disturbance which seemed to arise out of
wrestling matches between the citizens of
London and some men of the Abbot of Westminster. The first match was on the feast of
St James, the second on the day of St Peter
ad vincula. The sports ended in a riot and
strong men whom the steward of the Abbot

of Westminster had collected drove the Londoners into the city. The city bell was rung and in the presence of the Mayor, Serlo the mercer, a public meeting of the citizens was held. Serlo advised that compensation should be obtained from the abbot, but Constantine, son of Alulf, urged the destruction of buildings belonging to the abbot. These were probably on the abbey property near Cheapside and close to the place of meeting, so the exhortation was soon obeyed. Constantine shouted "Montjoie," the war-cry of the King of France. King Henry's friends were enraged and reported the affair to Hubert de Burgh, who sent into the city and ordered its seniors to appear before him. He asked them who dared to break the King's peace. Constantine said they had just cause. Hubert detained him and his nephew and one other in the Tower.

A charter of Constantine, son of Alulf, in

the cartulary of St Bartholomew's grants to
the hospital twenty shillings of annual quit
rent to support a priest who should say mass
three times a week for the salvation of Constantine's soul and that of his wife Katherine
and those of their children and for his ancestors and successors. The absence of the
usual witnesses of his time and with whom his
name so often appears suggests some unusual
circumstance in the time of granting this
charter. It is witnessed only by Gervase, a
priest, two citizens named Henry of St Helena
and Martin of Limoges, and its scribe, Richard
de Parmo. The charter ends with the words
"et aliis" instead of the usual "et multis aliis."
It may easily be imagined that it was written
on the anxious night in August which preceded
Constantine's execution. The morning after
the tumult, Hubert de Burgh, without any
trial, sent out the three prisoners with an

escort under Fulke de Breaute, who hanged them. Such was the end of Constantine, son of Alulf.

The brethren of St Bartholomew's in the next century witnessed another popular tumult. They saw Wat Tyler's mob in Smithfield, while Wat himself was dragged through the gate into the chamber of the master of the hospital. Sir Robert Knowles, an old combatant in the wars of Edward III and the Black Prince, was a tenant of the hospital in Smithfield, and rode out to protect King Richard on that day.

The next disturbed times with which the hospital had to do were those of the Great Rebellion.

The aspect of the hospital was more affected by war than it ever had been before. Colonels and captains sat on many committees of the governors and there were many

wounded soldiers in the wards. Letters were
sometimes read at the Court of Governors from
the Lord Protector, while the States arms, as
they were called, were prominent in the
Great Hall. Two soldiers who were patients
in a ward complained of the sister that she
used opprobrious and reviling speeches against
Sir Thomas Fairfax, namely, wishing his head
on London Bridge. She was formally re-
proved. The numerous soldiers and sailors
in the wards drank and quarrelled a
good deal. The King's execution, the Protector's death and Richard Cromwell's acces-
sion receive no mention in the Journals.
At a meeting on May 7, 1660, the treasurer
and seven governors being present, "It is
thought fit and ordered that the shield of
the States arms being the Red Cross and
Harp be taken down in the Great Hall and
the King's arms put in the room thereof."

On September 17 four names, one being that of Alderman Ireton, are ordered to be left out of the list of governors. Thus with as little clash as possible was royalty restored in St Bartholomew's.

A new steward was elected soon after the Restoration, and it was one of the recommendations of the successful candidate that he had fought bravely in the defence of Basing House. He proved a very excellent steward, and held office for a great many years.

Beds were reserved for eighty wounded seamen in the second Dutch war of Charles II. At the present day 200 beds are kept for wounded soldiers, while the staff also take charge of a large base hospital and are so closely employed that officers in uniform are even more numerous on the hospital paths than they were in the days of the Great Rebellion.

Such have been the occasional relations of St Bartholomew's to wars from the time of Magna Carta to our own days, in which it is giving shelter to many of our own wounded and those of our Belgian allies. During nearly eight hundred years it has continuously admitted as far as its rooms and means allowed all the sick and injured who have come to its doors.

At the present day Lazarus has as good food, nursing and treatment in the hospital as Dives has in his own house. The first step towards this essential condition of modern medicine at St Bartholomew's was the gift of William of Haverhill, sometimes called William son of Brithmar, who was sometime alderman of Cripplegate ward and was sheriff of London in 1189 and 1190. He gave during his lifetime and secured after his death fifteen shillings and two pence halfpenny to be spent each year in buying bread, so that every day there should be bought one ha'porth of white bread to be divided into eight parts to be given to the eight poor in the hospital who most needed it. The rest of the money was to remain as a provision in the kitchen on All Saints' Day for the use of the sick. The charter of William of Haverhill, though full of interest, is too long to read through to-day.

I fear I may have read too many charters already, but the past becomes so real in reading such documents that they have an extra-ordinary charm.

Addison in his essay on the effects of custom mentions how a great man known to him, who was no doubt Lord Somers, came to enjoy this study: "I have heard one of the greatest geniuses this age has produced, who had been trained up in all the polite studies of antiquity, assure me, upon his being

obliged to search into several rolls and
records, that notwithstanding such an employment was at first very dry and irksome to
him, he at last took an incredible pleasure in
it and preferred it even to the reading of
Virgil or Cicero."

When I began to write this lecture peace
reigned in Europe; before it was finished the
flames of war had begun to redden the sky.
At the time first appointed for its reading the
death in the field of my son Gillachrist, an
undergraduate of this University, prevented
it. Topics of war, and hardly any others,
interest us now, yet I have thought its subject
not unsuitable to the time, since the history
I have related tends to show how in a free
country such as ours, where everything is not
dominated by government, an ancient institu-
tion like St Bartholomew's Hospital, whether
in peace or war, lives with the nation and is

in touch with the national life in every period. The hospital is a field for the cultivation of knowledge, and great are the harvests which have been garnered thence since Harvey was its physician. It has the even greater duty of encouraging and maintaining the fraternal bonds which should exist throughout the nation between those who need help and those whose skill enables them to give it.

Its third function, which it shares with this University and all our other seminaries of sound learning, is the production of men, great even in their youth,

$$οἷοι νῦν βροτοί εἰσ'$$

as we may truly say, proudly reversing the Homeric use of the phrase. St Bartholomew's is not behind in this duty. It has sent more than a thousand such men into the field.

Milton Keynes UK
Ingram Content Group UK Ltd.
UKHW041519181024
449640UK00009B/74